PATHOLOGY

for kids

Medical School
FOR KIDS™

First paperback edition February 2024

Book design by Betty Nguyen & Brandon Pham

ISBN 978-1-957557-23-6 (paperback)

Printed in the United States of America

Published by Black Phoenix Press

www.mdforkids.org

To the friends and family who have supported and loved us unconditionally, and to the mentors who have guided and taught us more than we could have imagined:

Thank you.

Betty & Brandon

Medical School
FOR KIDS™

Pathology

(puh-THAA-luh-jee)

the branch of medicine concerned with the diagnosis of disease based on the microscopic examination of organs, tissues, and whole bodies

Medical School FOR KIDS™

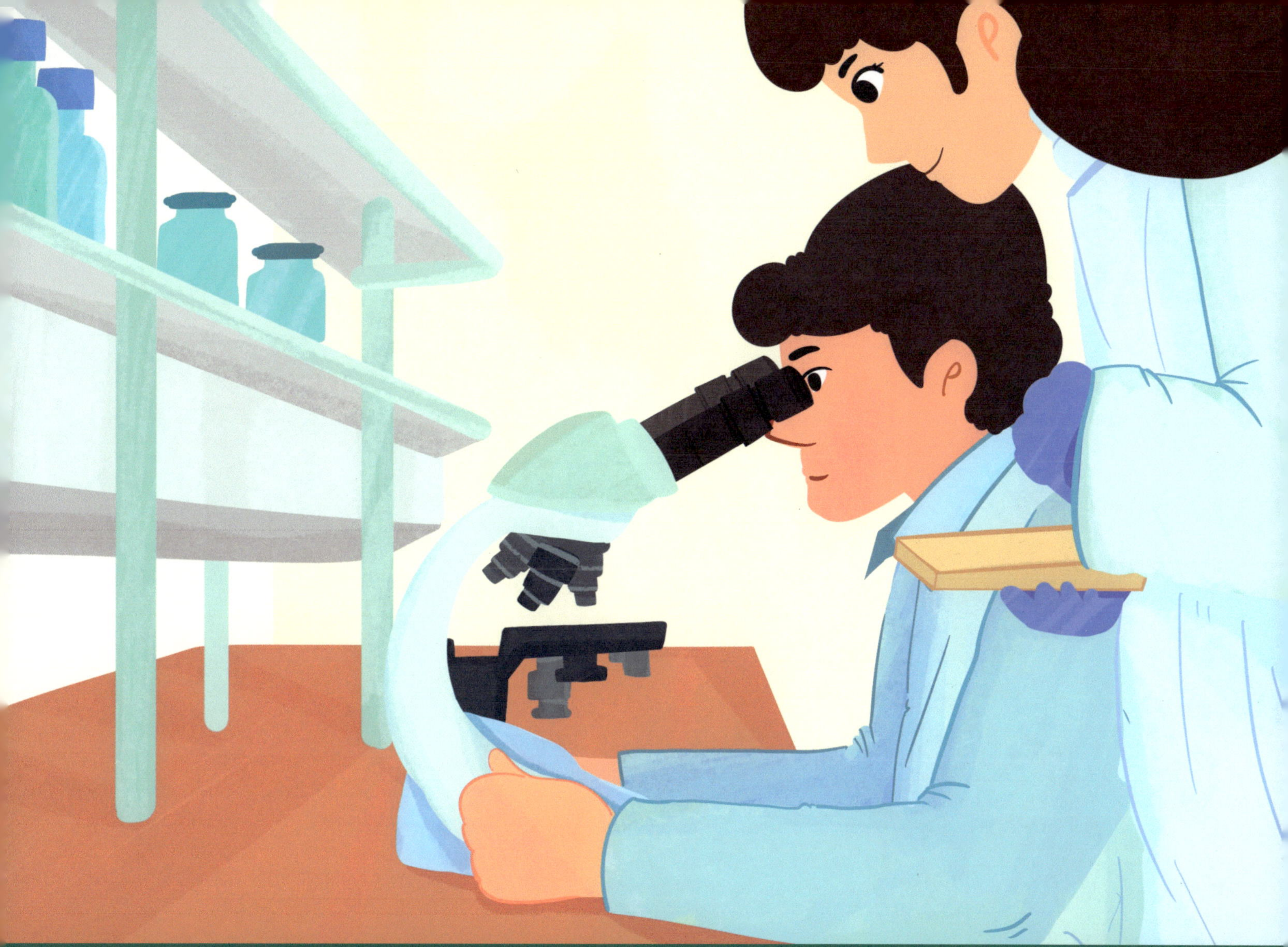

Pathologists are doctors who understand what's making people sick by looking at tiny samples of tissue from their bodies.

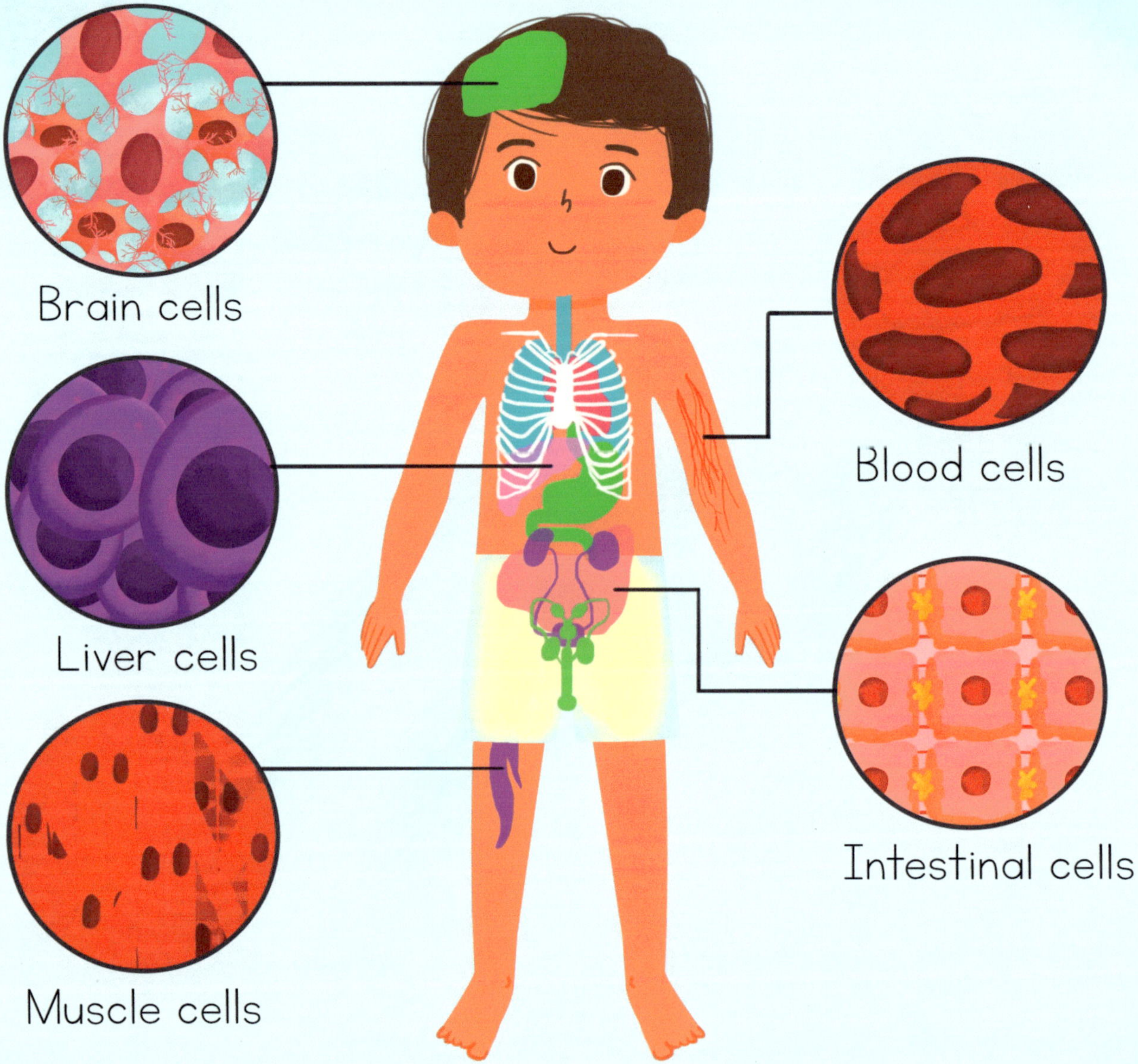

Body tissue is made up of **cells**, which are the basic building blocks of all living things.

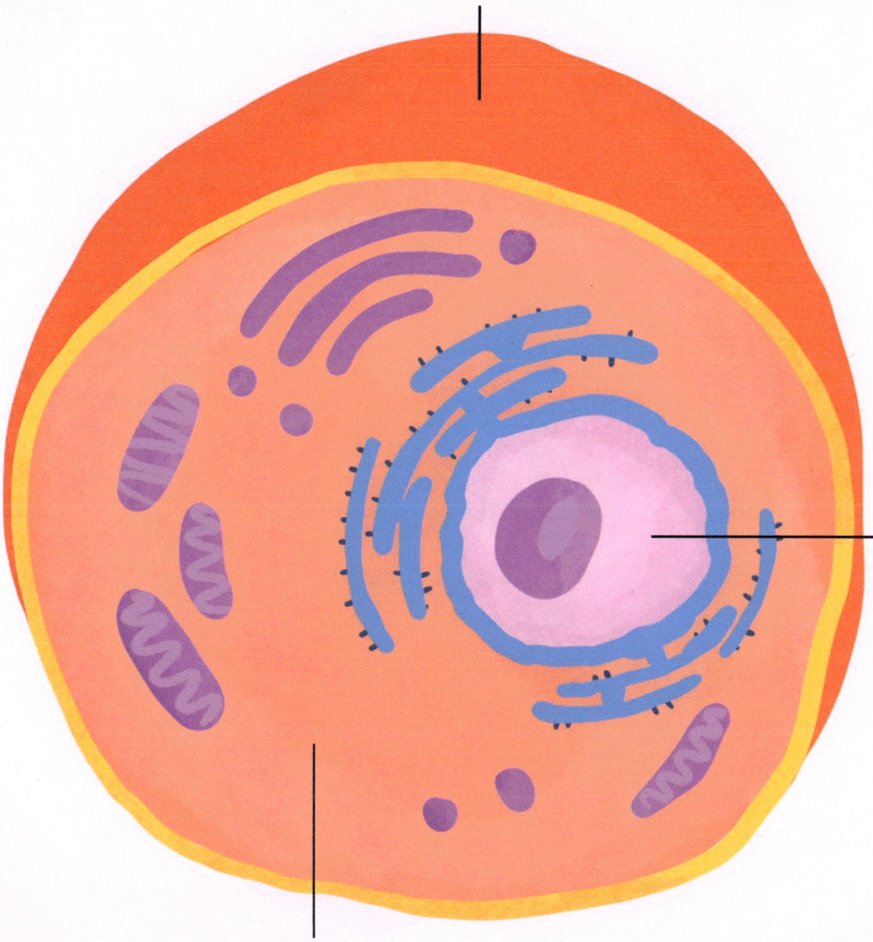

The three main parts of cells are the **nucleus**, **cytoplasm**, and **cell membrane**.

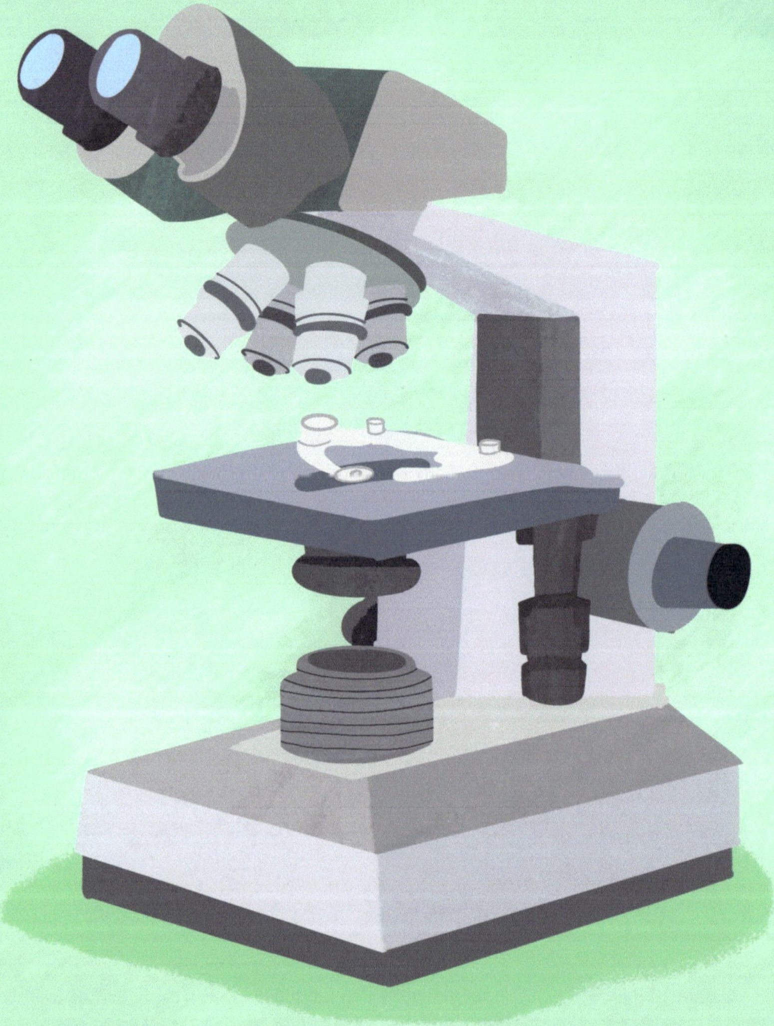

A **microscope** allows pathologists to see tiny details in cells and helps them understand what's happening inside our body.

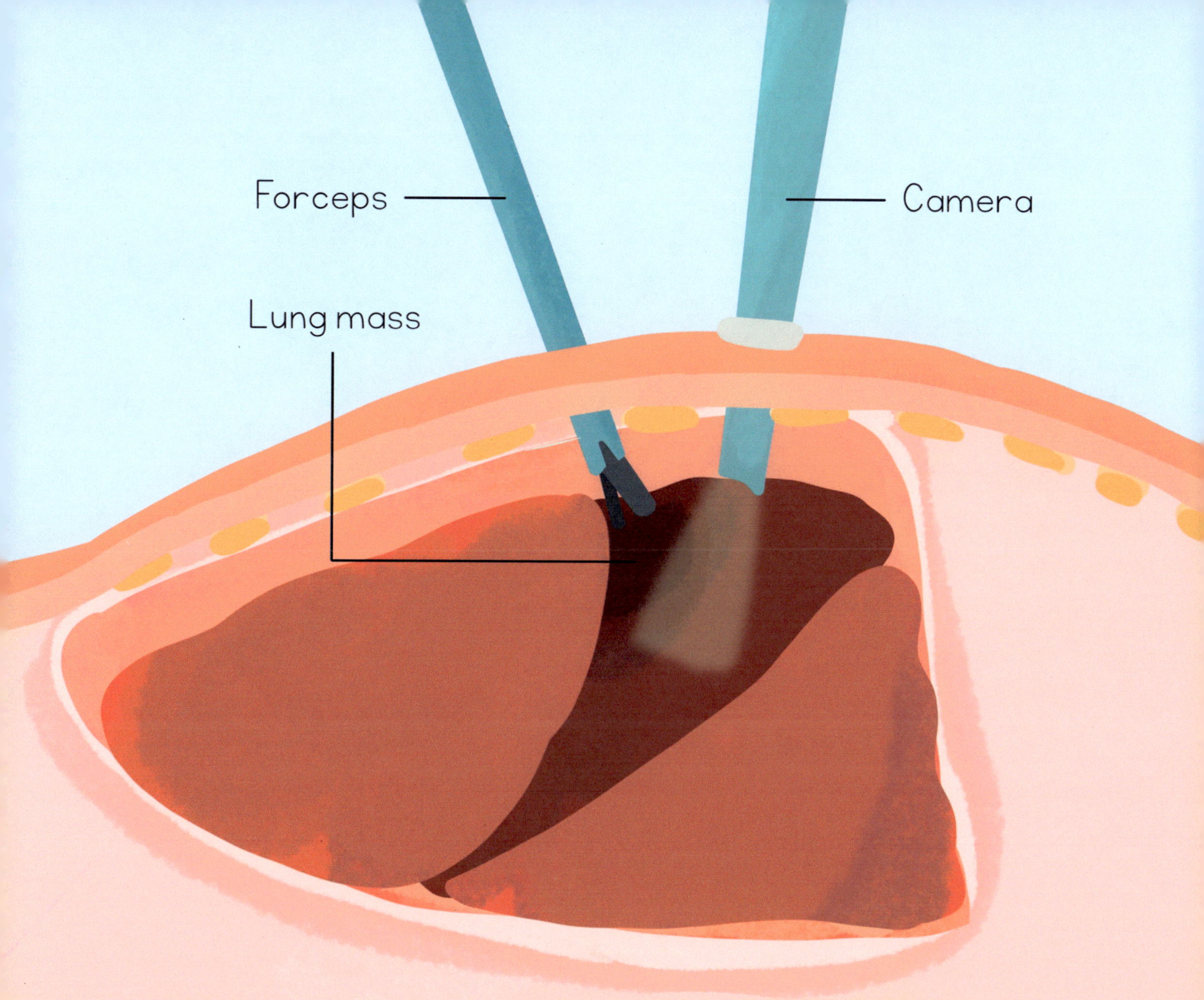

Samples of tissue are taken from the body through a procedure called a **biopsy**.

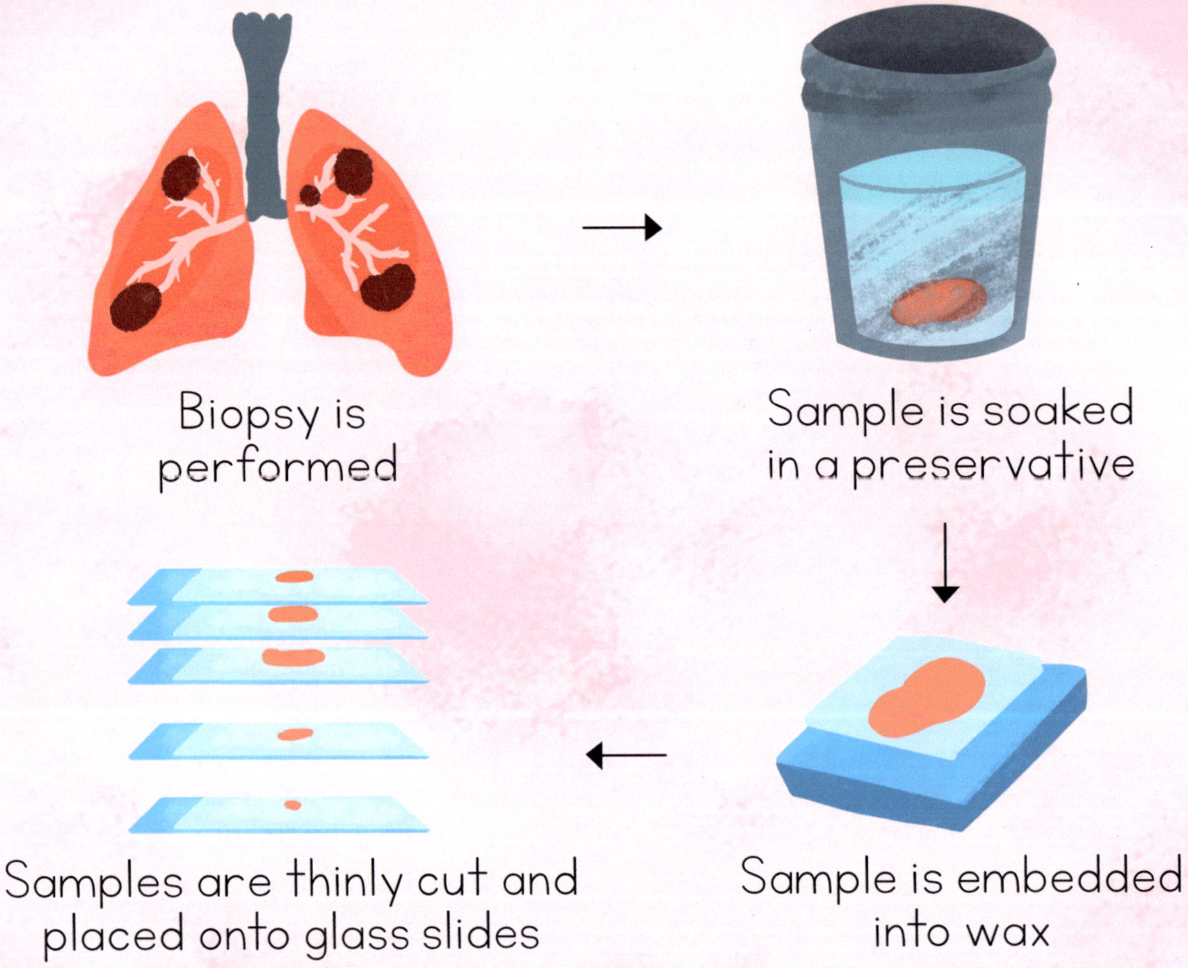

These samples are soaked in a preservative, embedded into wax, cut into thin sections, and placed onto glass slides.

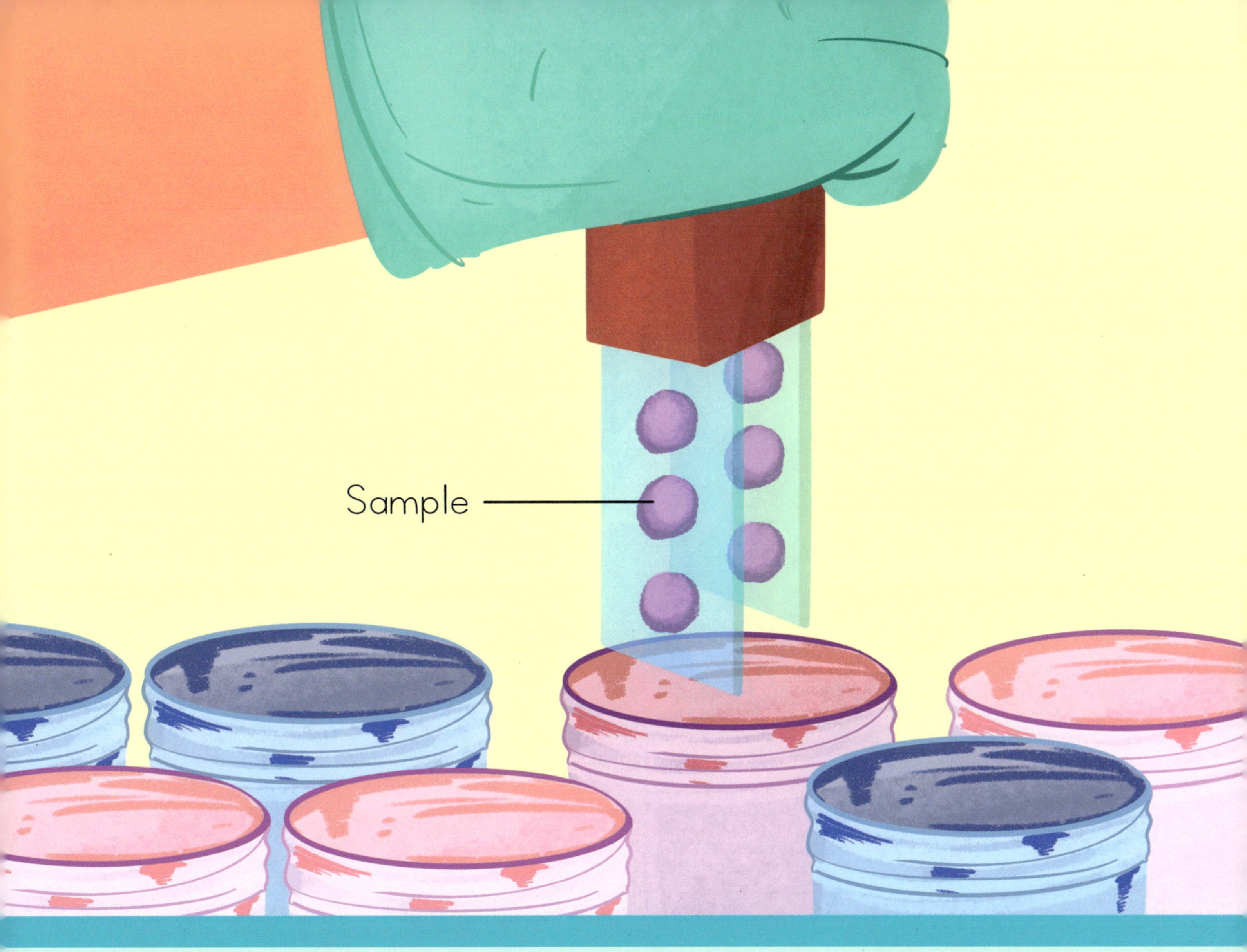

Special stains are used to color different parts of cells, which make them easier to identify under a microscope.

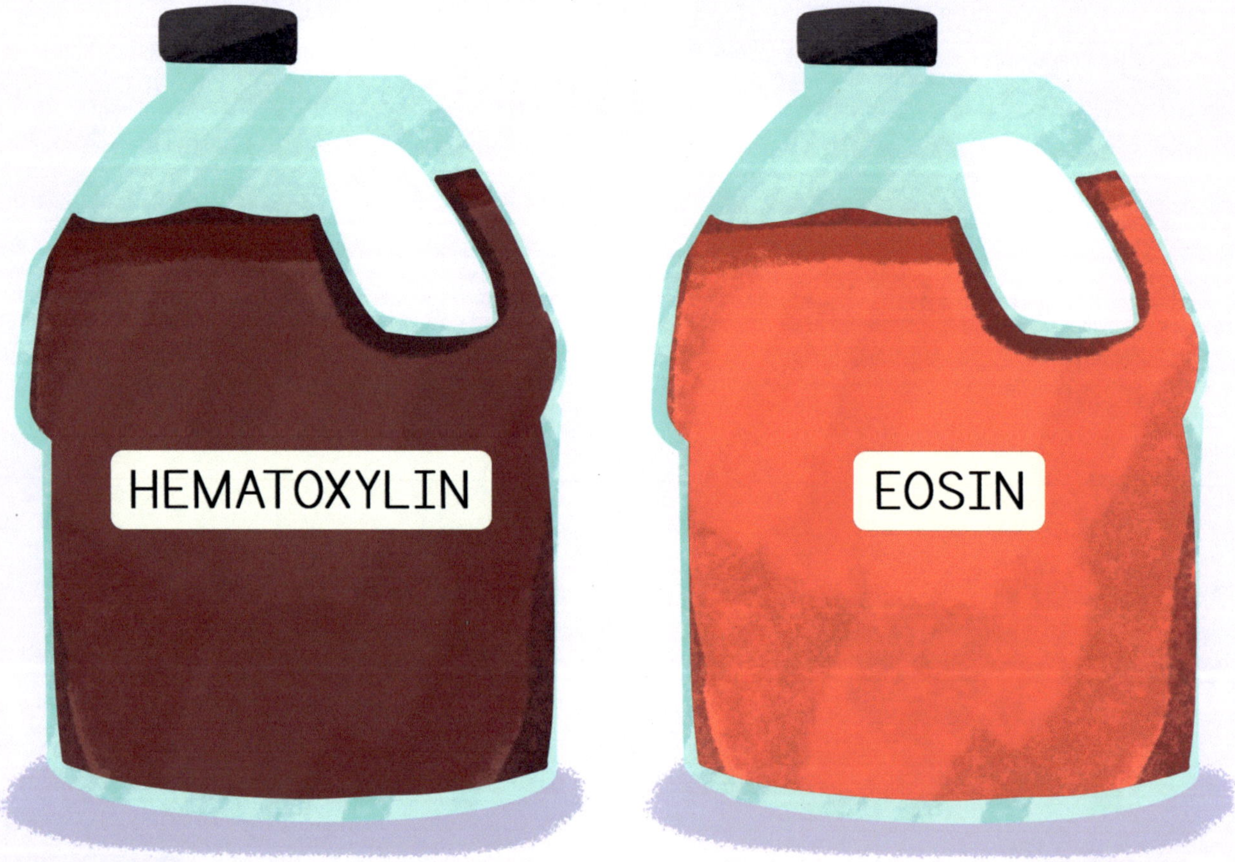

The most commonly used stain is the **hematoxylin and eosin (H&E) stain**.

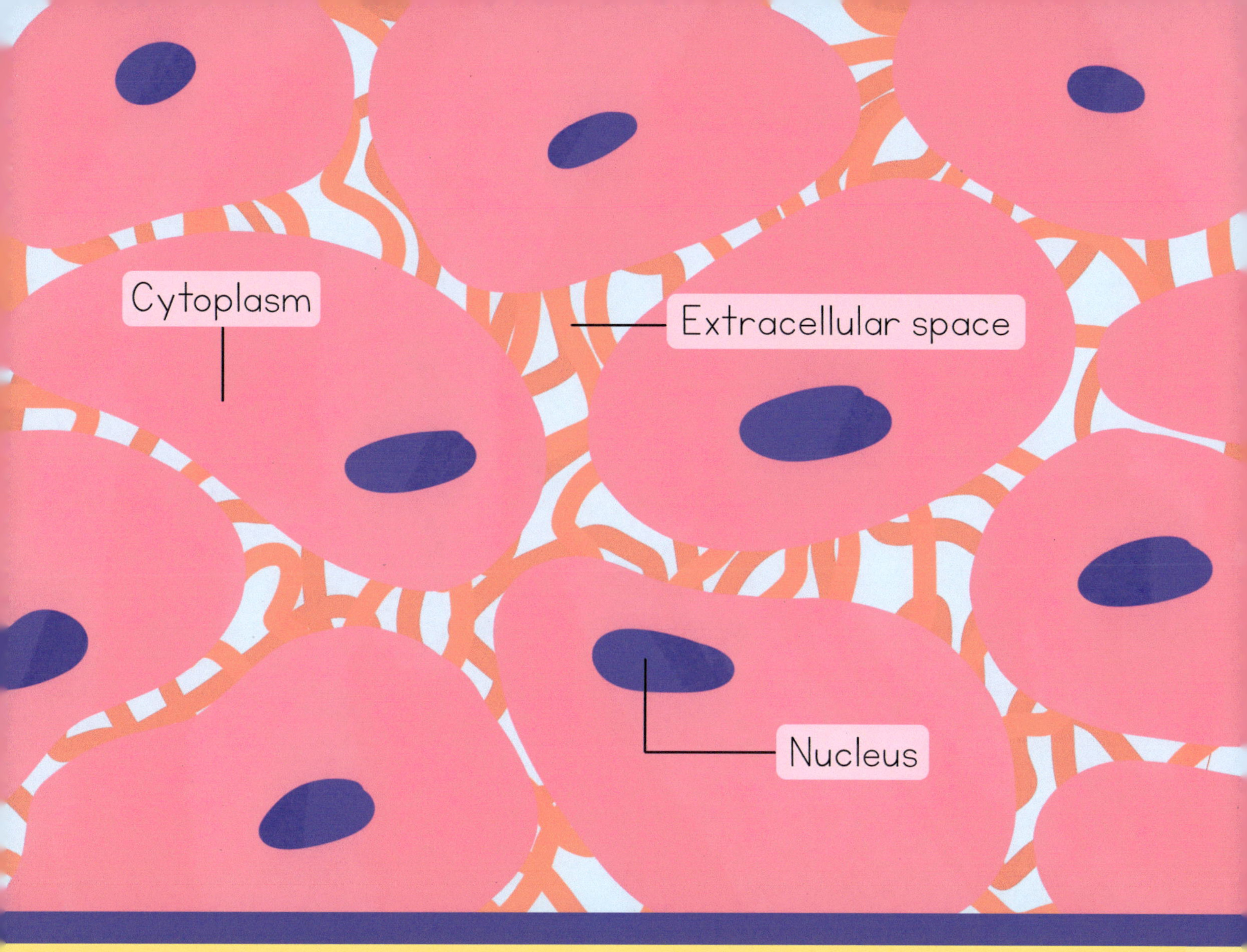

Hematoxylin stains the nuclei of cells *purple.*

Eosin stains the cytoplasm of cells and extracellular space *pink.*

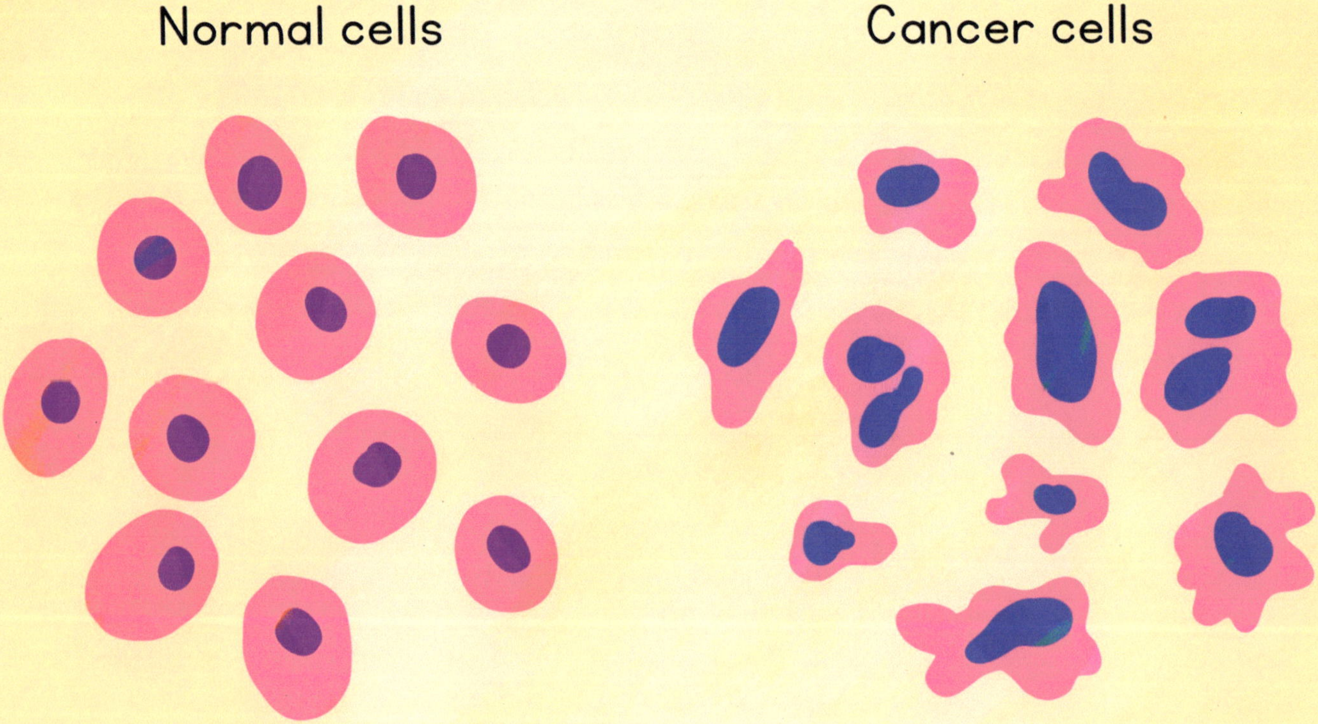

Diseases can affect how cells look under a microscope. Pathologists look for these changes to find out what's wrong.

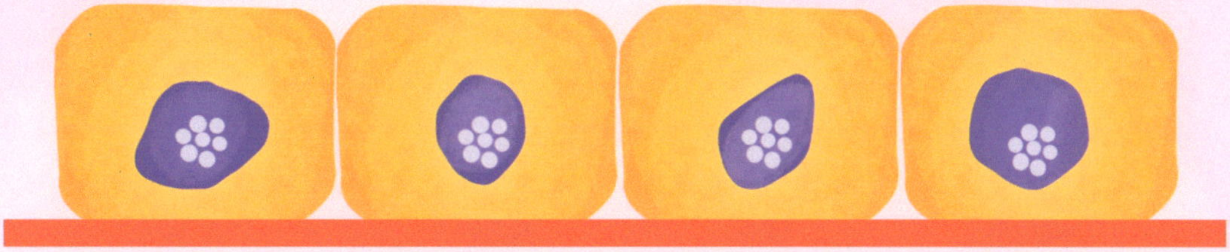

Normal cells

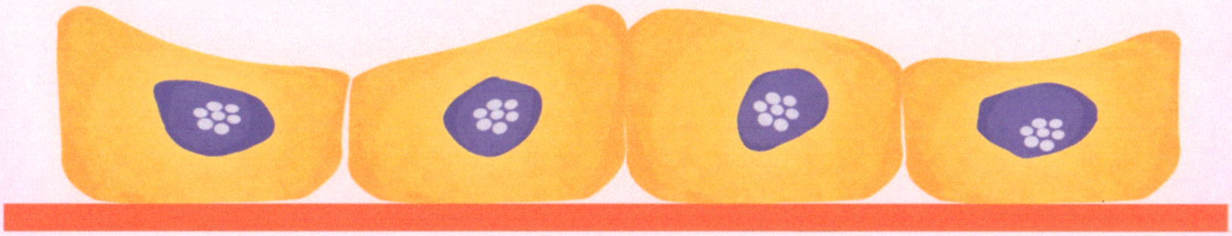

Atrophy

A decreased *size* of cells
is called **atrophy**.

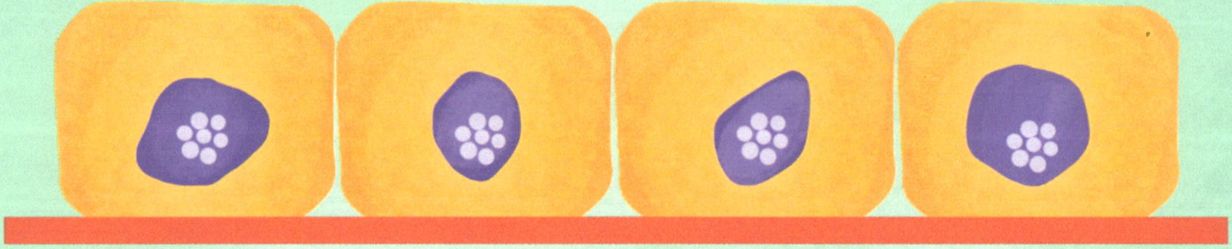

Normal cells

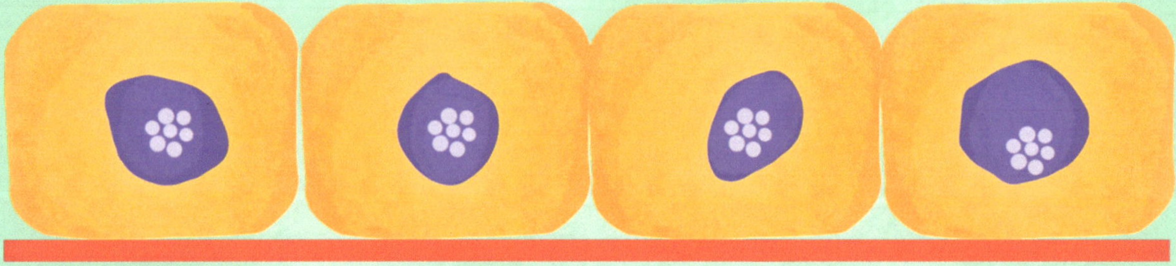

Hypertrophy

An increased *size* of cells
is called **hypertrophy**.

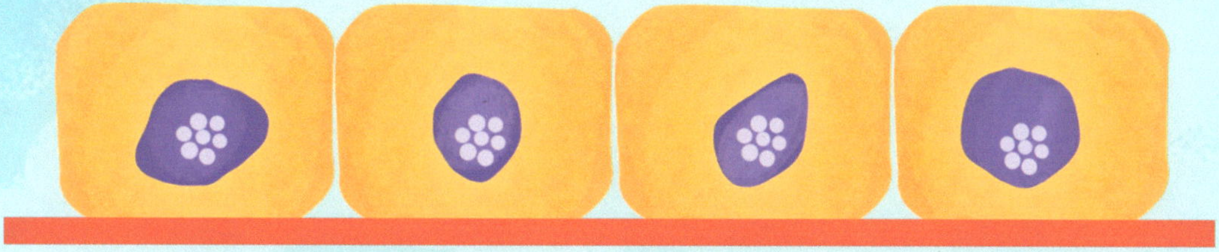

Normal cells

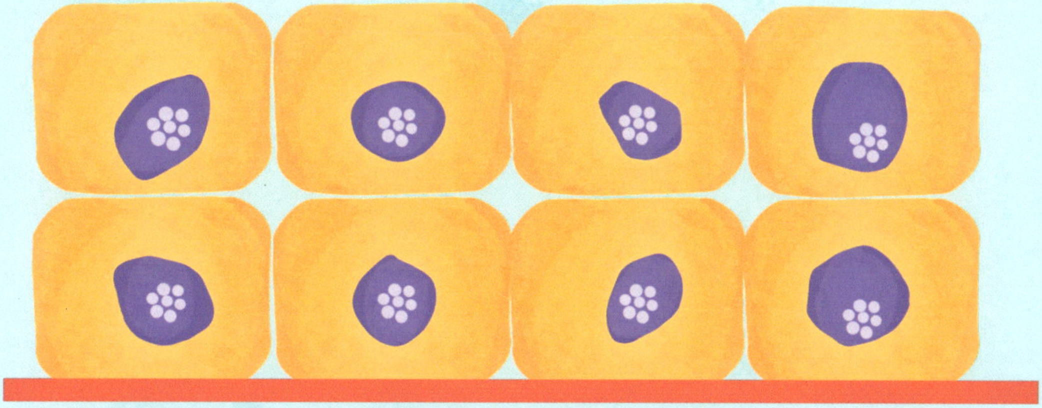

Hyperplasia

An increased *number* of cells
is called **hyperplasia**.

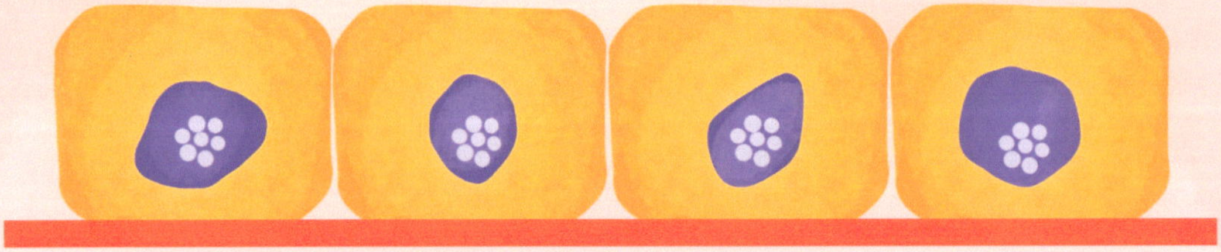

Normal cells

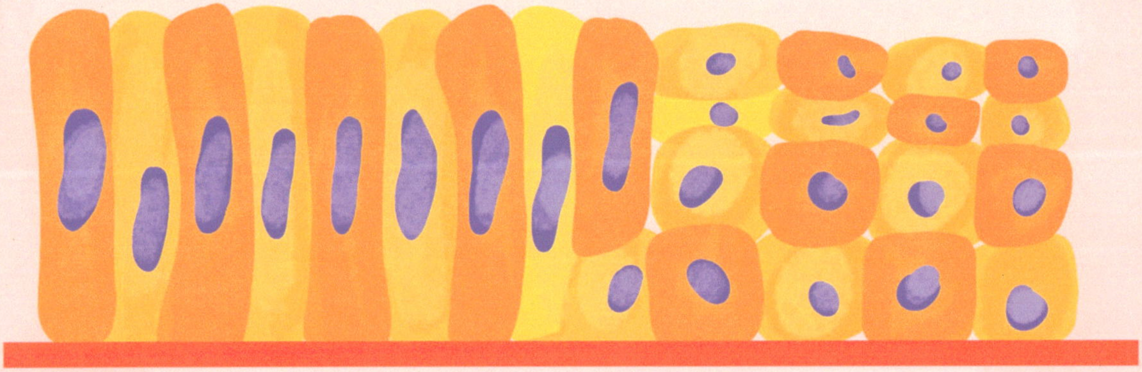

Metaplasia

The replacement of one cell type with another cell type is called **metaplasia**.

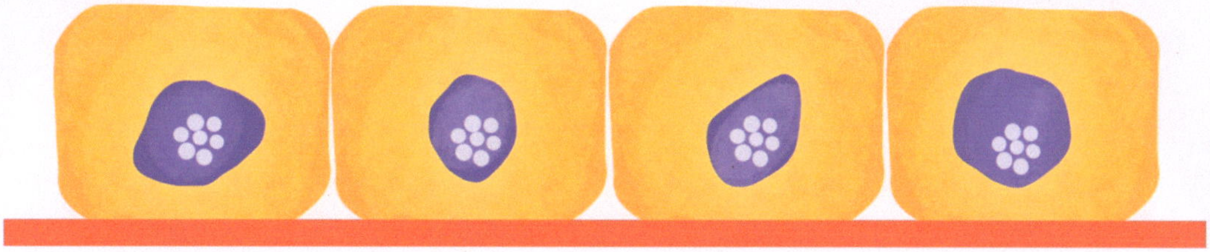

Normal cells

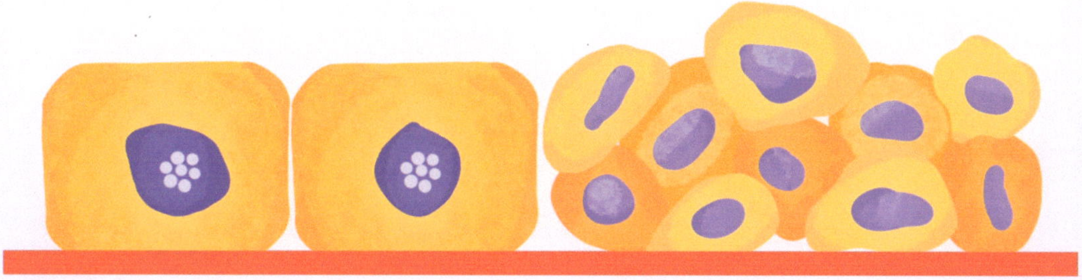

Dysplasia

The abnormal growth or development of cells is called **dysplasia**.

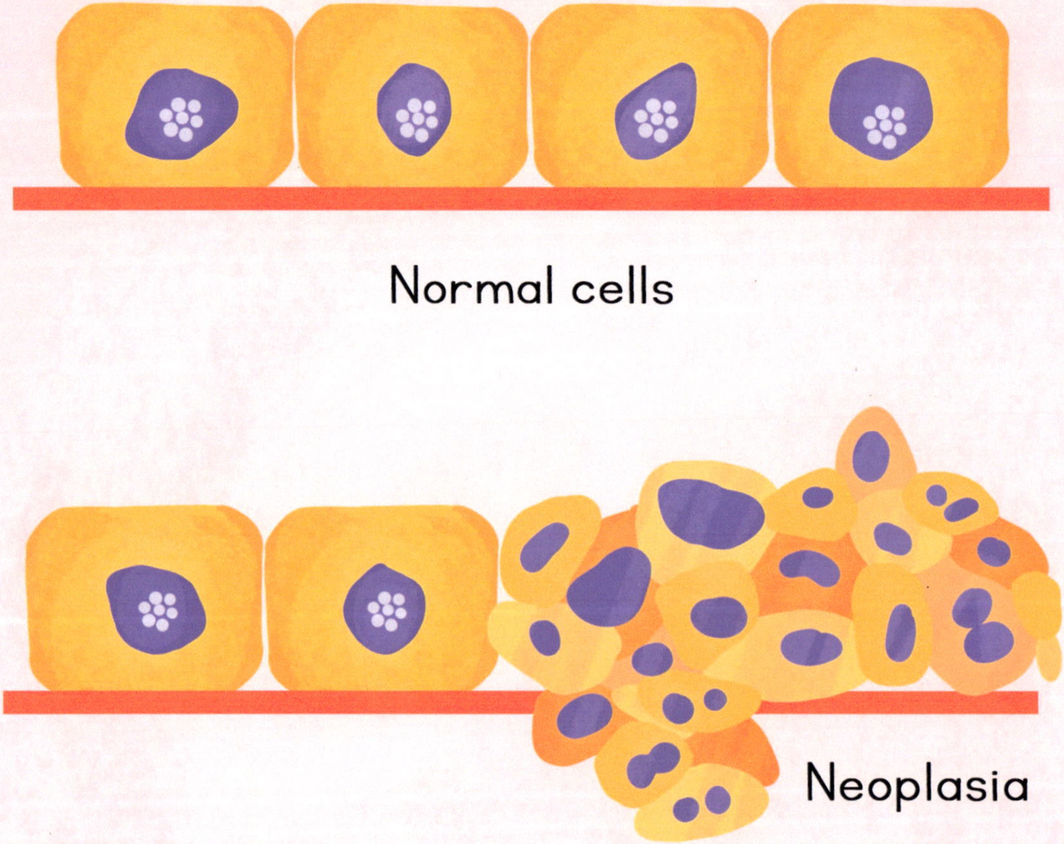

Sometimes, dysplasia can lead to **neoplasia**, which is the uncontrolled growth of cells that can form a **tumor**.

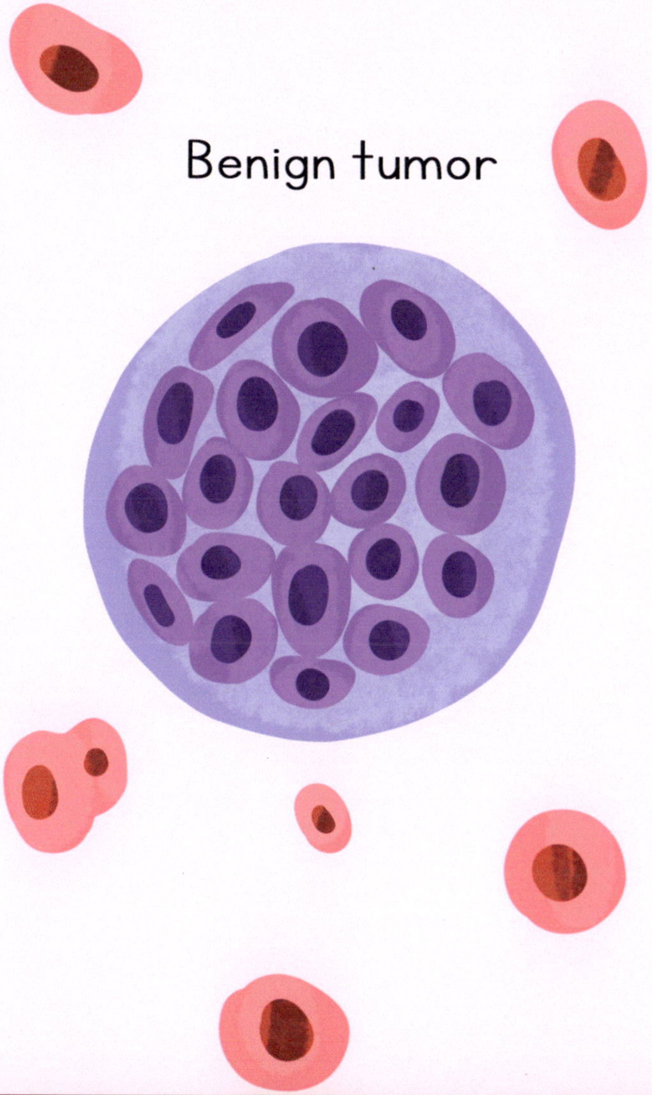

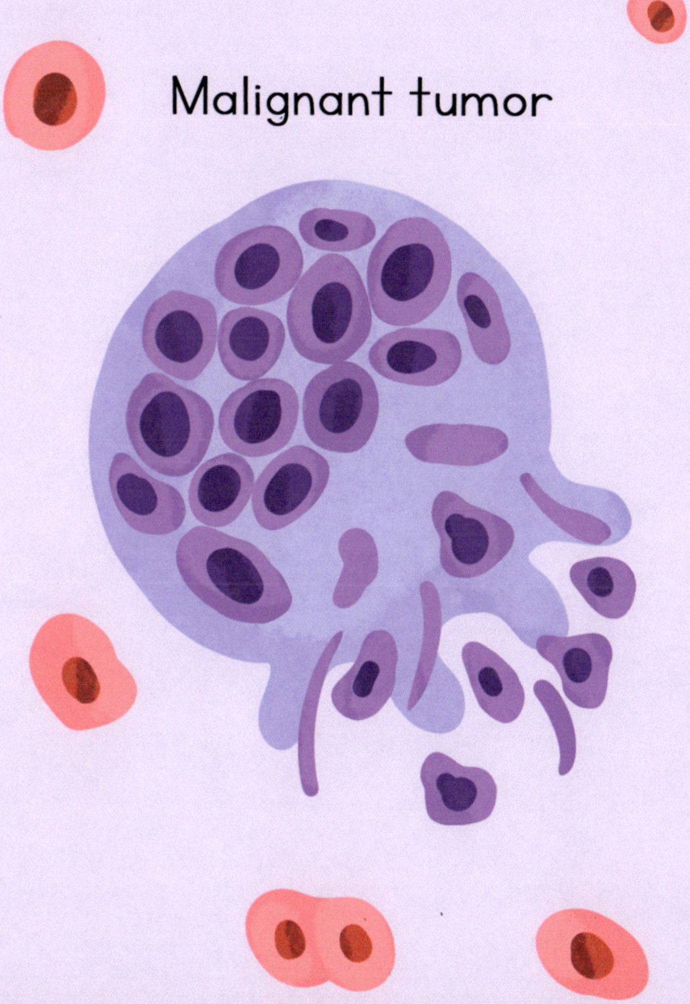

Benign tumors are non-cancerous.

Malignant tumors are cancerous.

Cancer can spread to other areas of the body.

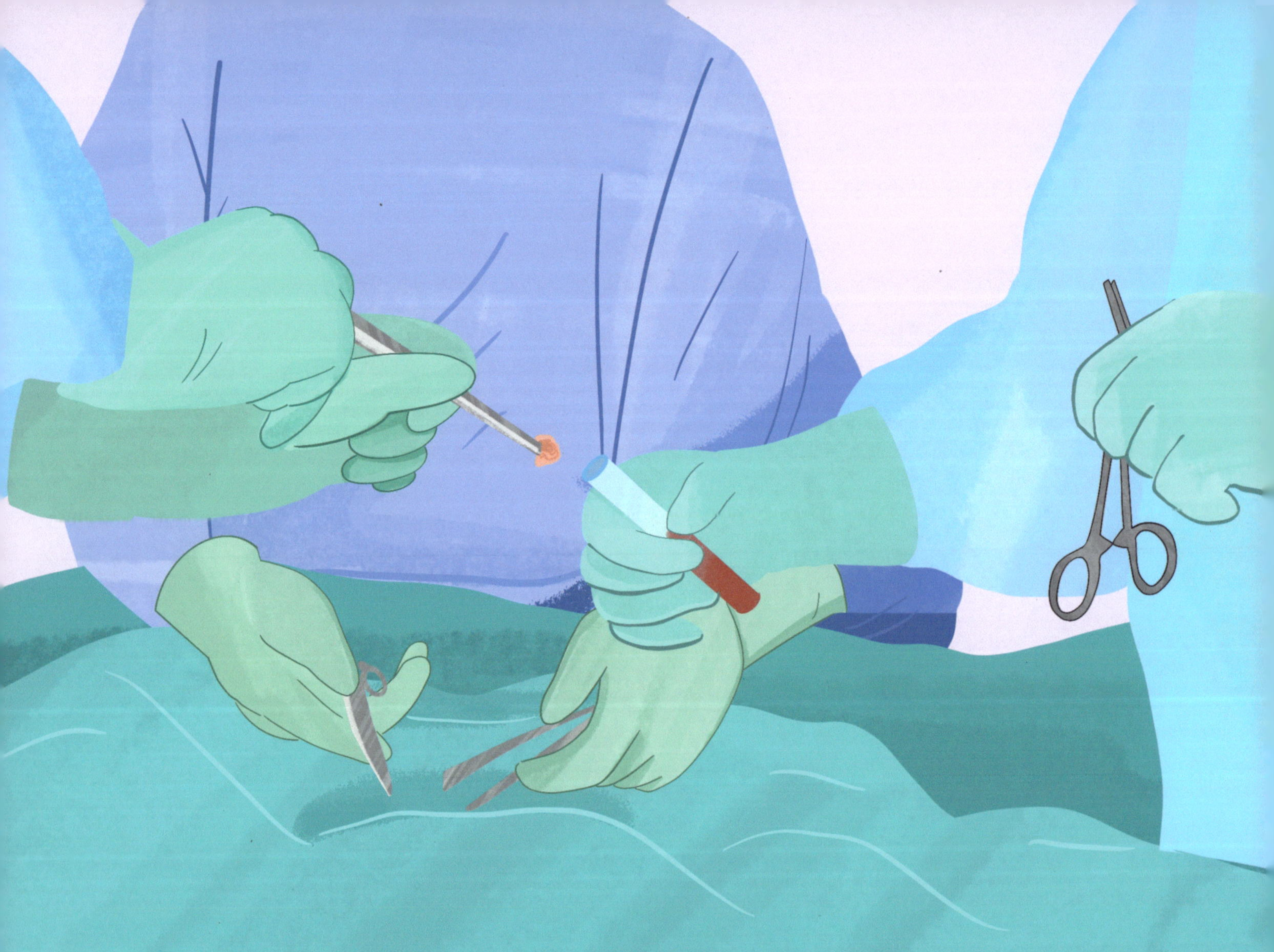

Sometimes during surgery, surgeons need to know whether tissue they are removing from a patient's body is cancer or not.

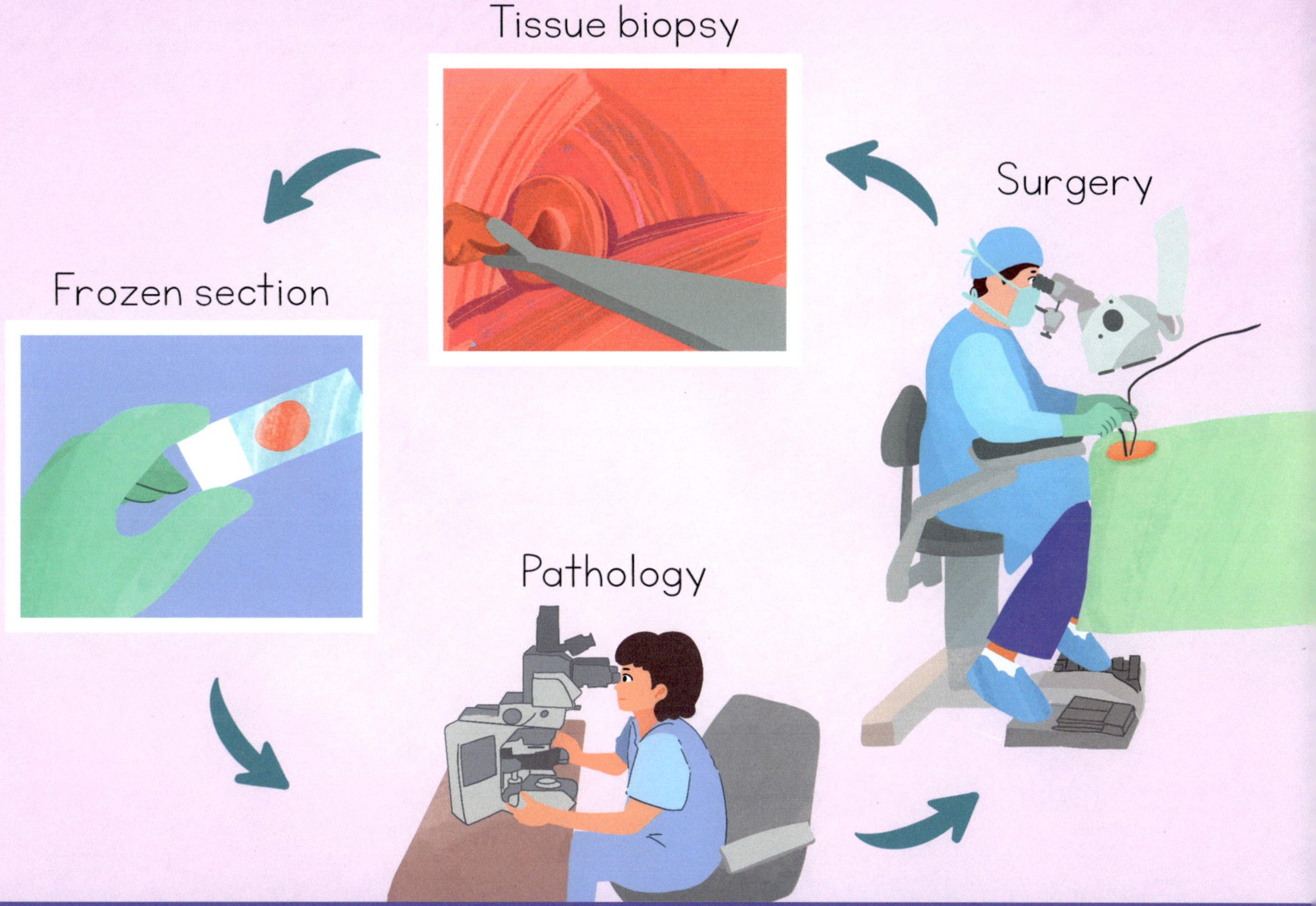

They can send special tissue samples, called **frozen sections**, to pathologists during surgery for rapid examination under a microscope.

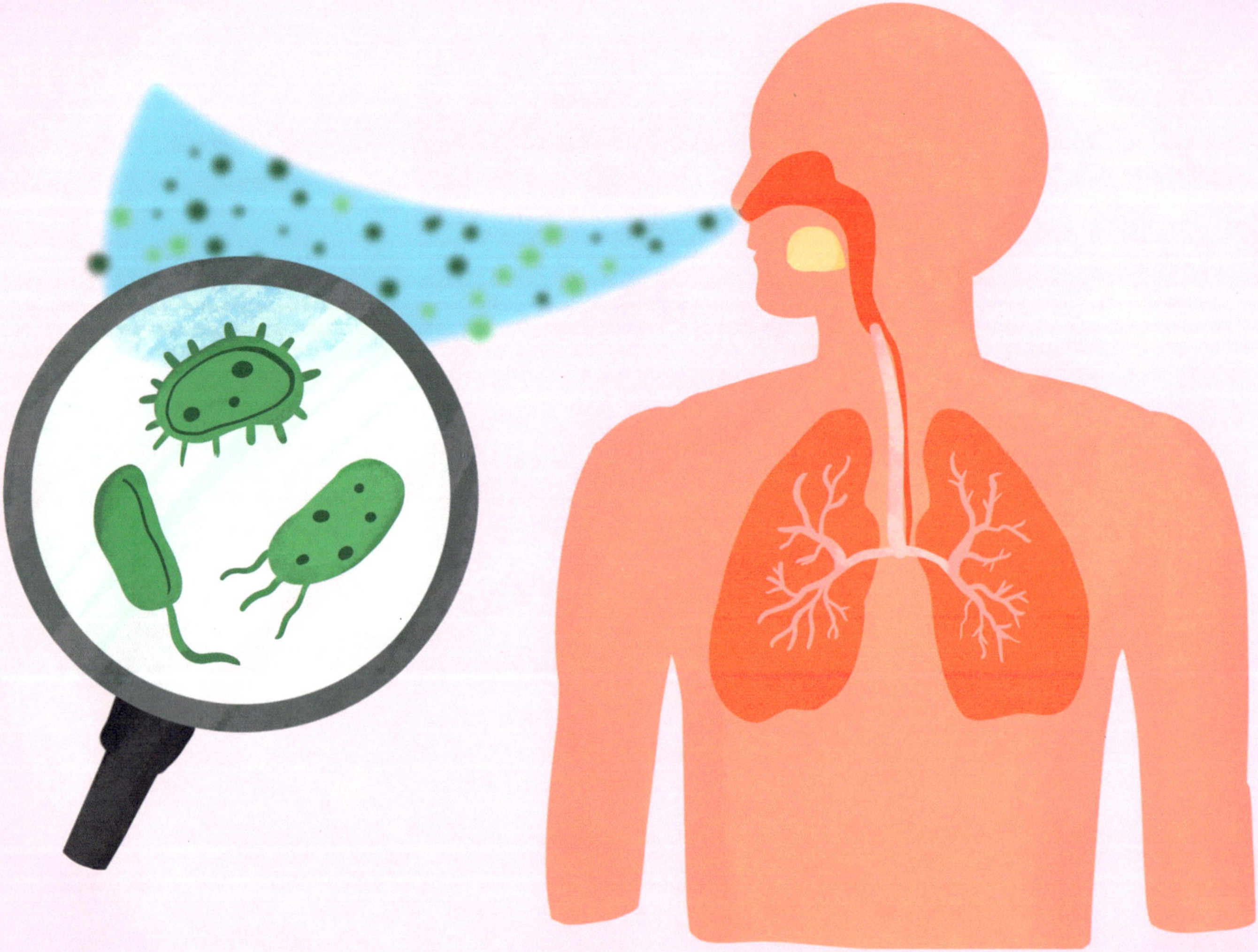

In addition to diagnosing cancer, pathologists diagnose **infections**, which occur when tiny microbes, such as bacteria, enter our body.

Steps of Gram staining

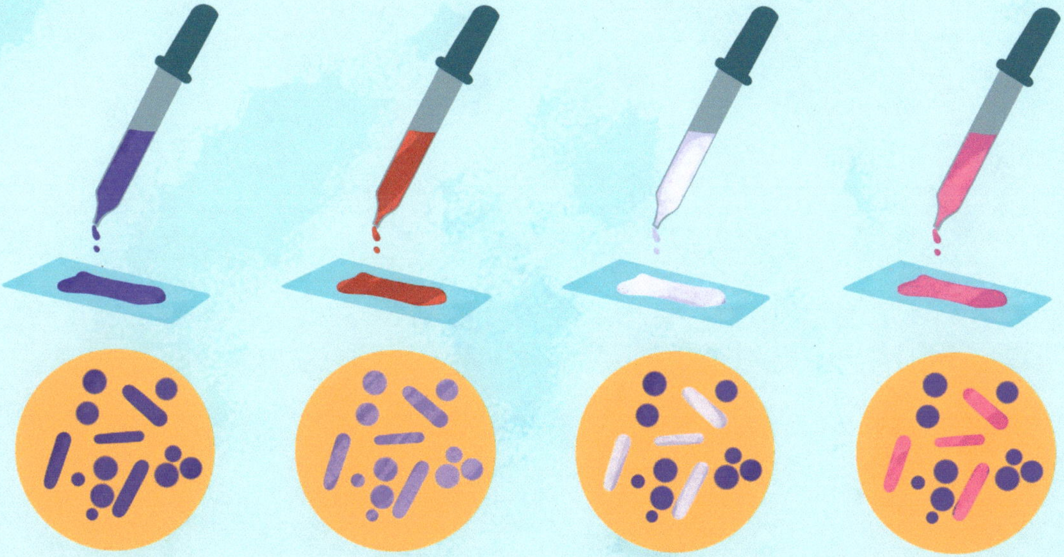

① Apply crystal violet
② Apply iodine
③ Alcohol wash
④ Apply safranin

A special type of stain that helps identify bacteria in tissue samples is called a **Gram stain**.

Gram-negative bacteria

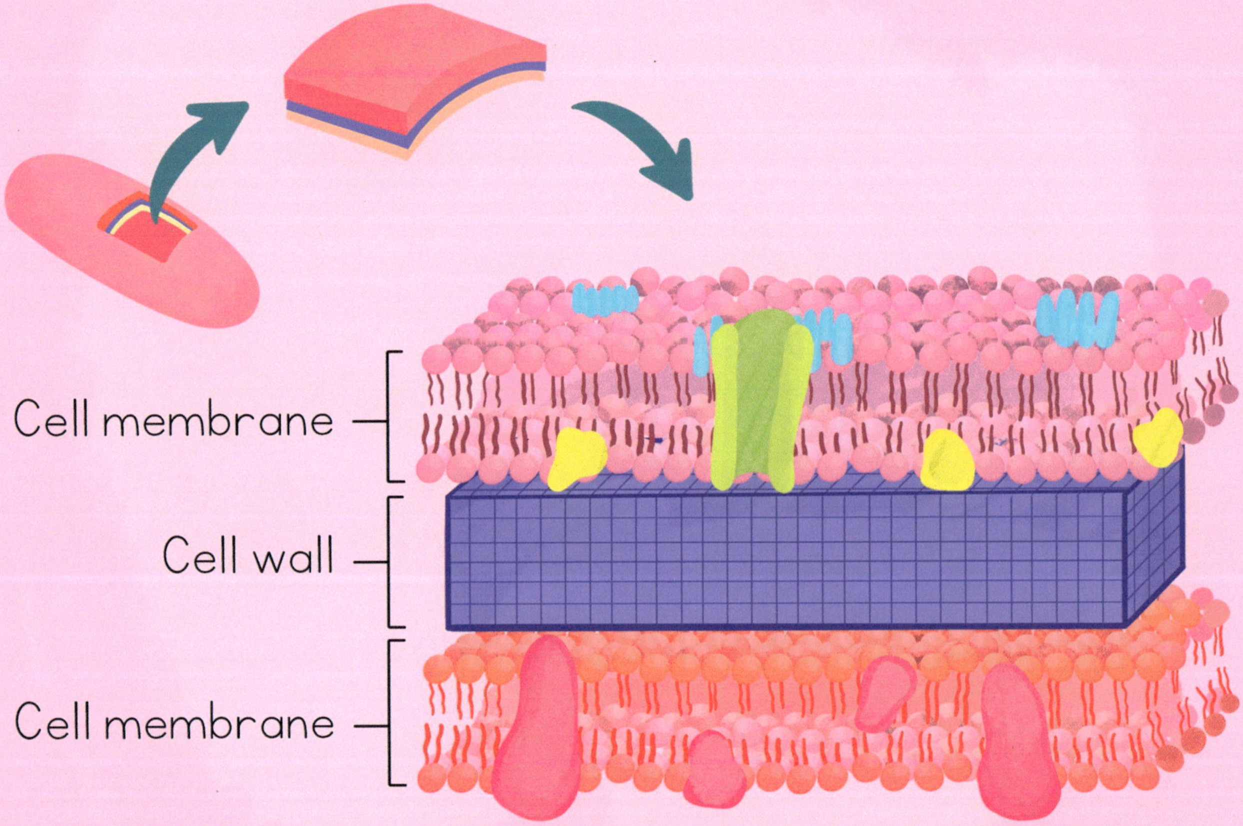

Gram-negative bacteria appear *pink* after Gram staining. They have a *thin* cell wall surrounded by an outer cell membrane.

Gram-positive bacteria

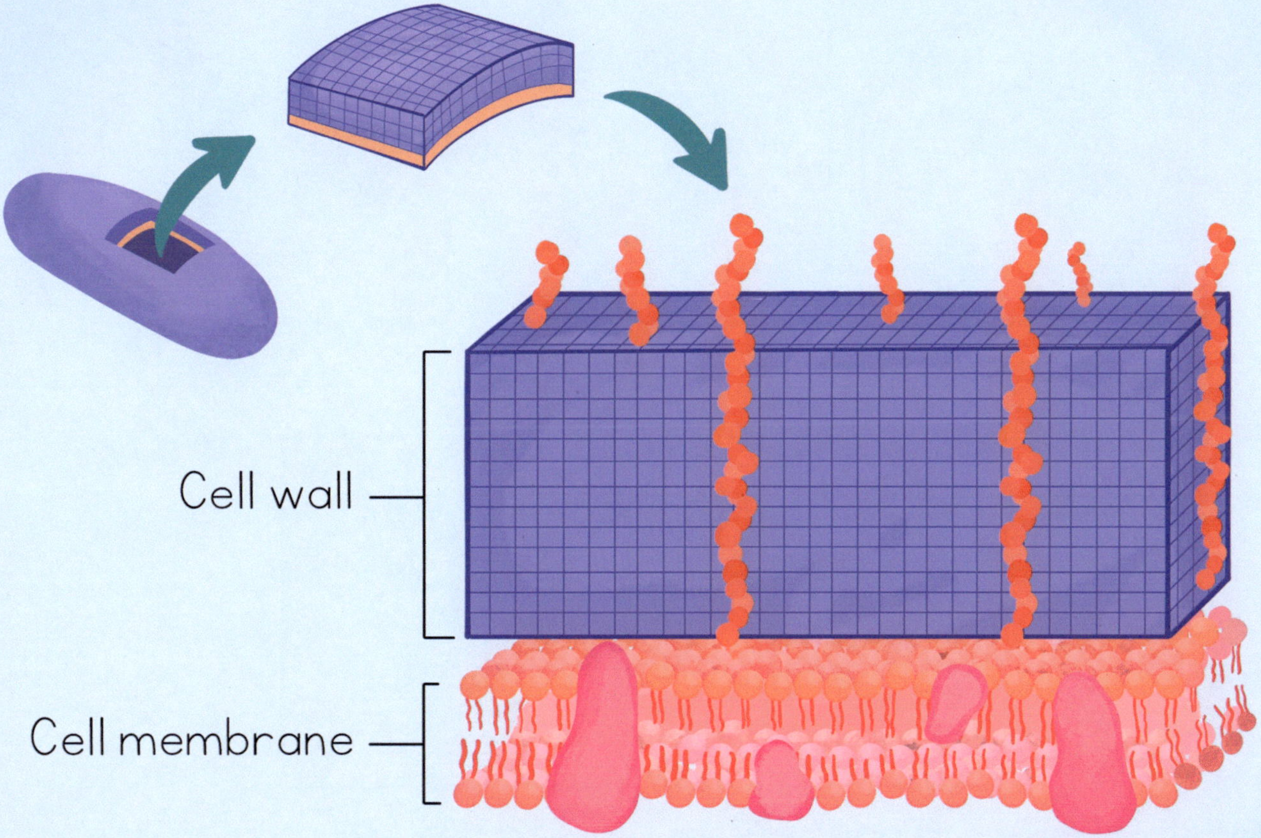

Gram-positive bacteria appear *purple* after Gram staining. They have a *thick* cell wall and *no* outer cell membrane.

Types of leukocytes

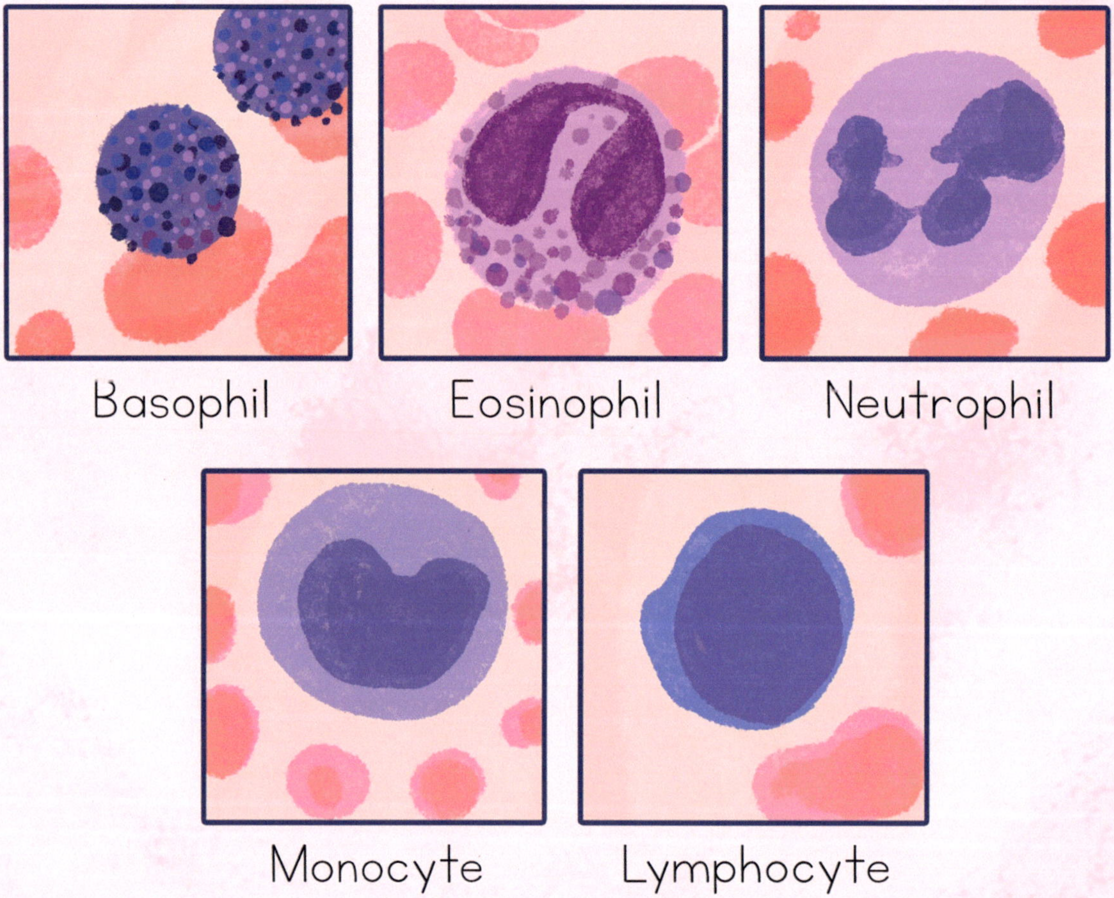

Inflammation occurs when **leukocytes**, or white blood cells, travel to sites of infection. There are many types of leukocytes!

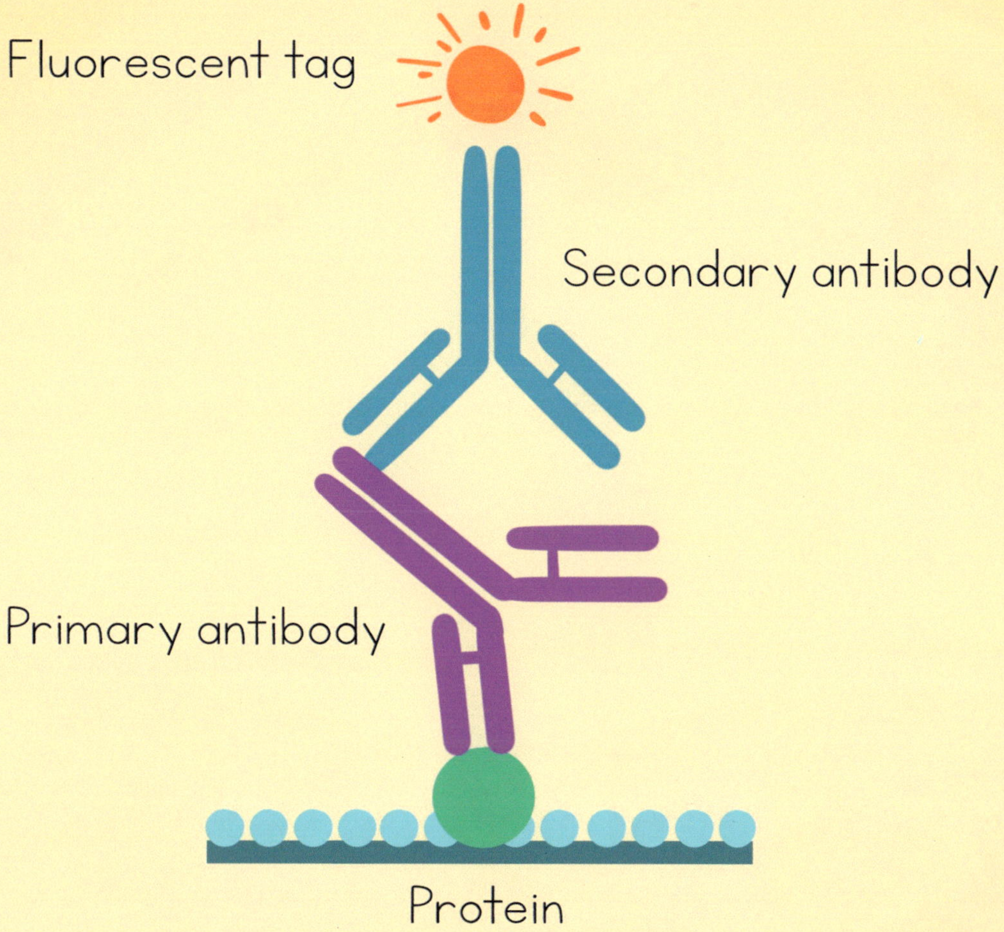

Pathologists can identify specific proteins in tissue using antibodies that find the protein and light up! This is called **immunohistochemistry**.

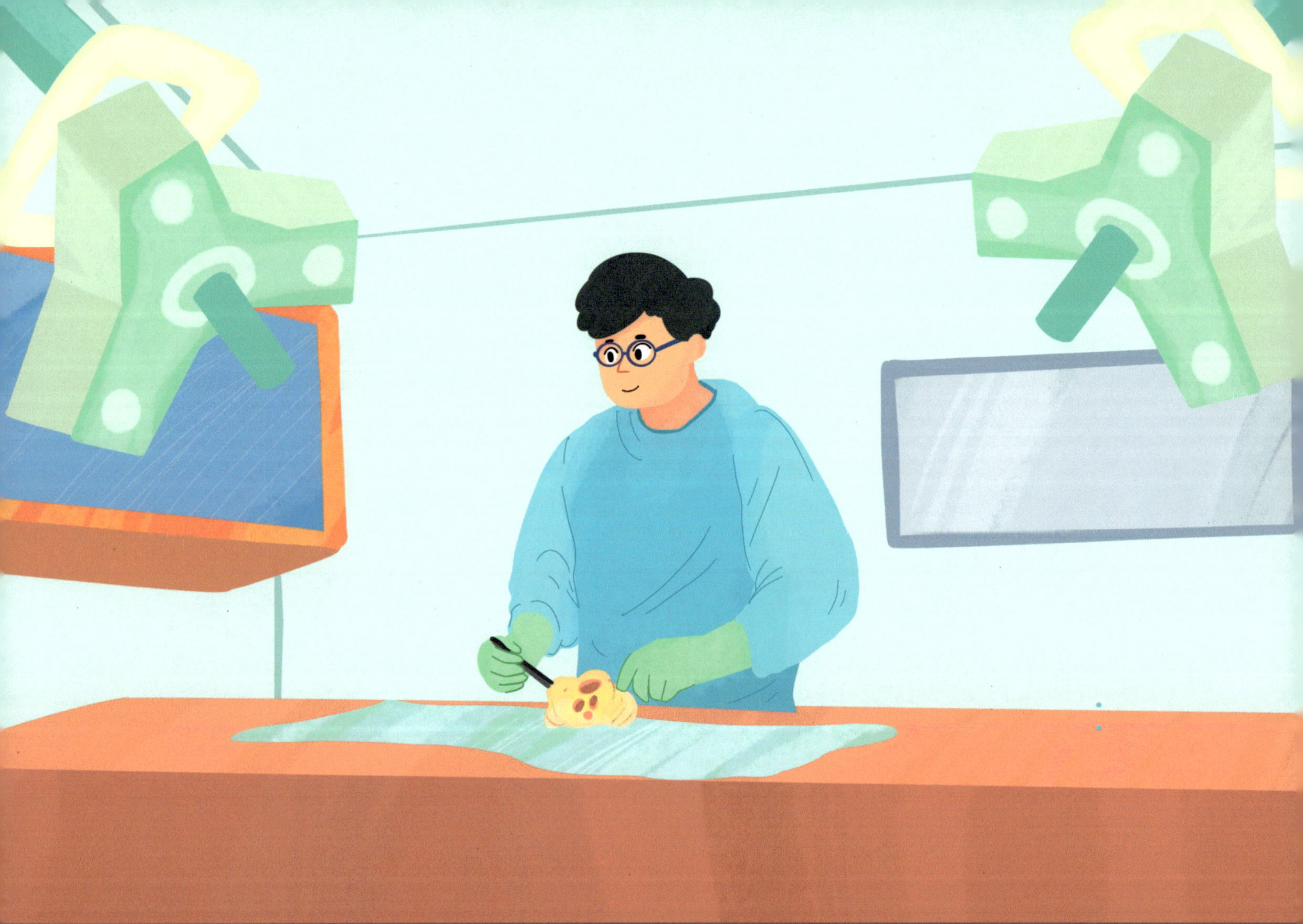

Forensic pathologists specialize in performing **autopsies**, which can determine the cause of a person's death.

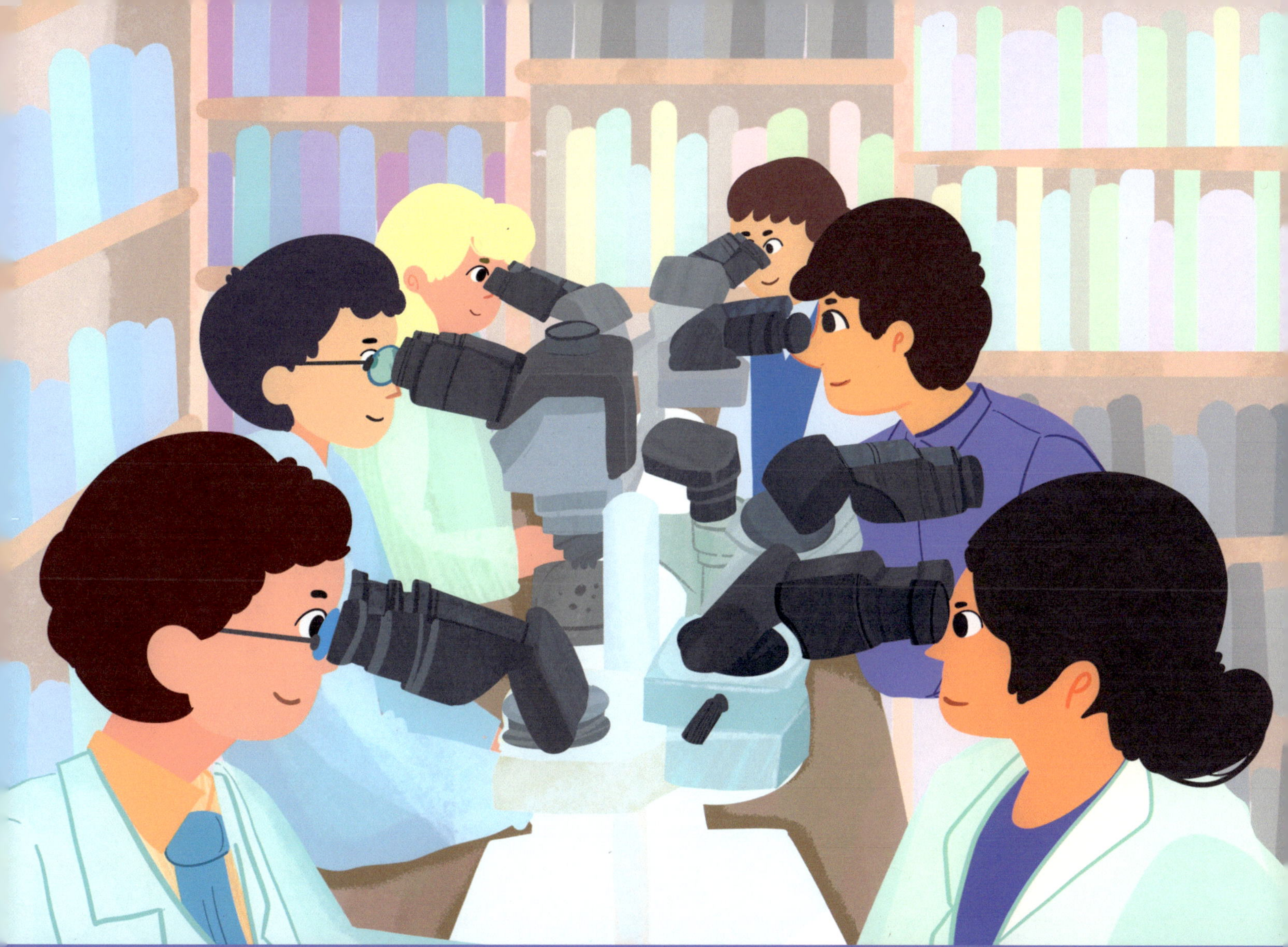

Pathologists always work on a team. They look at specimens under a microscope to diagnose medical problems and help other doctors treat patients.

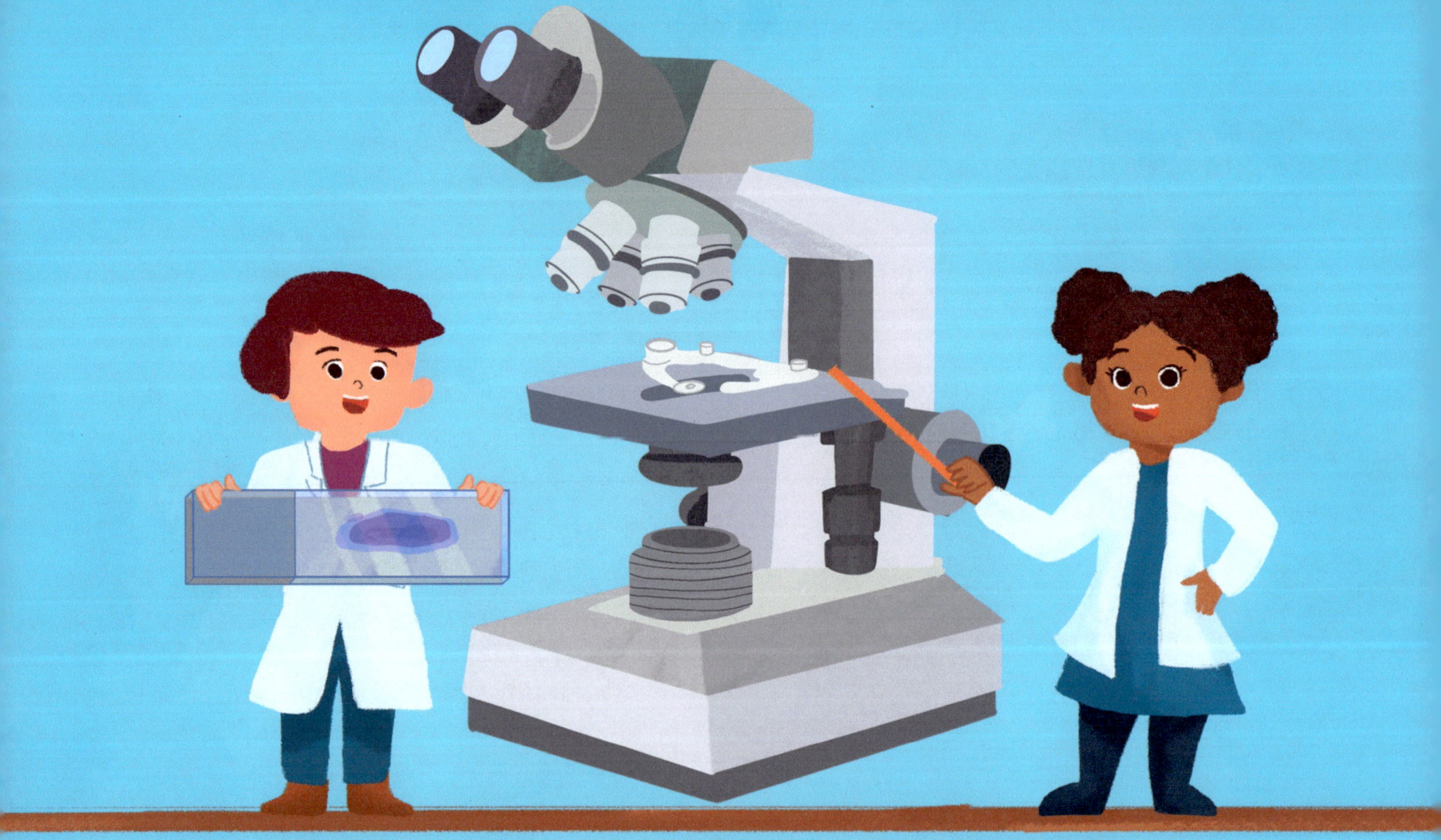

YOU'RE A FUTURE PATHOLOGIST!

Glossary

Atrophy (AH-truh-fee): decrease in size of cells

Biopsy (BAI-aap-see): removal of samples of tissue or cells from the body

Cell (sel): smallest unit of an organism that is the building block of living things

Dysplasia (dis-PLAY-zhuh): abnormal growth or development of cells

Eosin (EE-uh-sn): dye that stains cell cytoplasms pink

Forensic pathologist (fr-EN-zuhk puh-THAA-luh-juhst): type of pathologist who performs **autopsies**, which can determine the cause of a person's death

Frozen section: procedure in which tissue is frozen and thinly sliced for evaluation under a microscope; guides surgeons in real-time during surgery

Gram stain: method of staining used to distinguish between **gram-negative** (pink) and **gram-positive** (purple) organisms

Hematoxylin (hee-muh-TAAK-suh-luhn): dye that stains cell nuclei purple

Hyperplasia (hai-pur-PLAY-zhuh): increase in number of cells

Hypertrophy (hai-PUR-truh-fee): increase in size of cells

Immunohistochemistry (im-yuh-noh-hiss-toh-KEM-uh-stree): lab technique that uses antibodies to find and attach to certain types of proteins on cells

Infection (in-FEK-shn): condition caused by microbes that enter the body; can trigger **inflammation**, or recruitment of white blood cells (**leukocytes**)

Metaplasia (meh-tuh-PLAY-zhuh): replacement of one cell type with another

Microscope (MAI-kruh-skowp): instrument used to see very small objects

Neoplasia (nee-oh-PLAY-zhuh): uncontrolled growth of cells that can form a **tumor**; can be **benign** (non-cancerous) or **malignant** (cancerous)

Let's review what you learned!

1. What are the three main parts of cells?
2. What instrument do pathologists use to look at cells?
3. What is the name of the procedure in which samples of tissue are taken?
4. What dye is used to stain the nucleus of cells purple? What dye is used to stain the cytoplasm pink?
5. What is a decreased size of cells called? Increased size of cells?
6. What is an increased number of cells called?
7. What is the replacement of one cell type with another called?
8 What is the abnormal growth or development of cells called?
9. What is the uncontrolled growth of cells that can form a tumor called?
10. What type of tumor is non-cancerous? What type of tumor is cancerous?
11. What type of tissue samples can surgeons send to pathologists for rapid examination and diagnosis during surgery?
12. What special stain helps identify bacteria in tissue samples?
13. What color do gram-positive bacteria and gram-negative bacteria appear after Gram staining?
14. What is the process by which leukocytes travel to sites of infection called?
15. What lab technique uses antibodies to identify specific proteins in tissues?
16. What type of pathologist specializes in performing autopsies?

Your Answers

1. ______________________
2. ______________________
3. ______________________
4. ______________________
5. ______________________
6. ______________________
7. ______________________
8. ______________________
9. ______________________
10. ______________________
11. ______________________
12. ______________________
13. ______________________
14 ______________________
15. ______________________
16. ______________________

Medical School FOR KIDS™

Answer Key

1. Nucleus, cytoplasm, and cell membrane
2. Microscope
3. Biopsy
4. Hematoxylin; eosin
5. Atrophy; hypertrophy
6. Hyperplasia
7. Metaplasia
8. Dysplasia
9. Neoplasia
10. Benign; malignant
11. Frozen sections
12. Gram stain
13. Pink (gram-negative); purple (gram-positive)
14. Inflammation
15. Immunohistochemistry
16. Forensic pathologist

Medical School FOR KIDS™

About the Authors

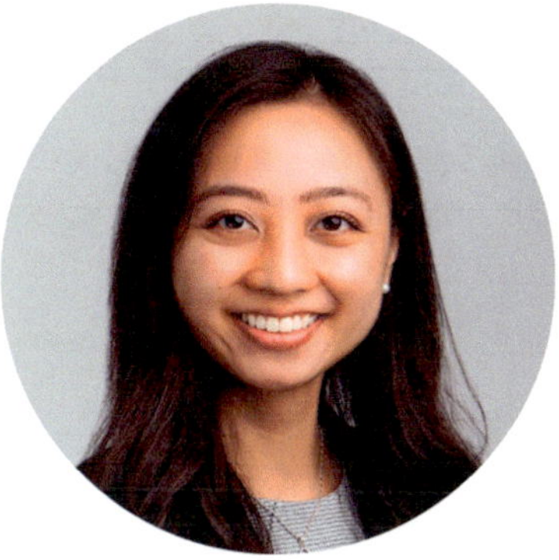

Betty Nguyen, MD

Betty is a physician specializing in dermatology. She was born in California but spent much of her childhood in Georgia, where she grew up on a chicken farm. Betty studied Biology at UCLA, where she was a Gates Millennium Scholar, and earned her MD from UC Riverside on a full-tuition scholarship. Outside of work, Betty is a certified yoga instructor and licensed scuba diver. She also enjoys journalistic writing and cycling.

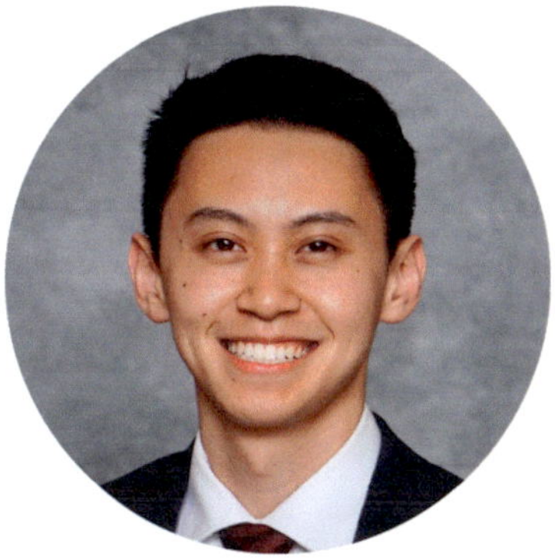

Brandon Pham, MD

Brandon is a physician specializing in ophthalmology. He was born and raised in California. Brandon studied Microbiology, Immunology, and Molecular Genetics at UCLA, where he was a Barry Goldwater Scholar, and earned his MD from Stanford. He is passionate about medical education for students of all ages. In his free time, Brandon enjoys traveling, playing tennis, and performing card magic tricks.

Medical School FOR KIDS™

Check out the rest of the books in our series!

Website: mdforkids.org

Instagram: @md.for.kids

Medical School
FOR KIDS™